CUPPING THERAPY

A Comprehensive Guide To Discover The Ancient Art Of Cupping, Harnessing Its Healing Power To Relieve Pain, Reduce Stress, And Revitalize Your Body And Mind

WILFREDO CARSON

INTRODUCTION

Cupping therapy, also known as hijama or suction therapy, is an ancient medicinal technique that has been used for millennia in many cultures. This treatment includes applying suction to the skin using cups made of glass, bamboo, or silicone. Cupping therapy is thought to improve blood circulation, relieve tension, and aid in the body's natural healing processes. This article will go over the history, purpose, benefits, and different types of cupping techniques, providing a thorough explanation of this traditional therapy.

<u>A brief overview of cupping therapy:</u>

Cupping therapy originated in traditional medical systems such as Traditional Chinese

Medicine (TCM), Ayurveda, and Middle Eastern medicine.

Cupping is based on the notion of creating a vacuum on certain parts of the body using either heat or suction.

This vacuum action raises the skin and underlying tissues, boosting blood circulation, lymphatic drainage, and the movement of vital energy, also known as qi or prana in various cultures. Cupping therapy is frequently used in conjunction with acupuncture, massage, and other holistic treatments to address a variety of health concerns.

<u>Historical Background:</u>

Cupping therapy dates back thousands of years, with evidence found in ancient

Egyptian, Chinese, and Middle Eastern civilizations.

Cupping has been described in Chinese medicine from 1550 BCE, according to the Ebers Papyrus, one of the earliest medical textbooks in existence.

Cupping therapy is referenced in the Hadith, or sayings and actions of Prophet Muhammad, indicating that it was used in the seventh century. The Greeks also embraced cupping, with Hippocrates, often considered the father of Western medicine, approving the procedure for a variety of conditions.

Cupping therapy has evolved and been incorporated into a wide range of cultural and medical traditions throughout history.

It regained prominence in the West in the nineteenth century and is still practiced today,

pg. 5

both in traditional settings and by modern healthcare experts looking into complementary and alternative therapies.

<u>Purpose and Benefits of Cupping Therapy:</u>

Cupping therapy is used for a variety of objectives, including pain relief and relaxation, as well as treating specific health concerns.

The primary goal is to improve blood circulation and eliminate stagnation in the body's energy channels. This is said to promote the body's natural healing mechanisms, improving overall health. Cupping is frequently used to relieve musculoskeletal discomfort, such as back and neck pain, by relaxing muscles and increasing blood flow to the affected areas.

The therapy is also said to cleanse the body by promoting the evacuation of metabolic waste and toxins via the lymphatic system. Cupping, according to traditional Chinese medicine, is supposed to balance the body's essential energy, resolving imbalances that might cause illness. Cupping therapy is also used to promote respiratory health because it is thought to relieve congestion and improve lung function.

Cupping therapy has benefits that go beyond the physical, with many practitioners and clients experiencing improved mental and emotional well-being.

Cupping can generate relaxation, which can reduce tension and anxiety while also promoting a sense of equilibrium. While scientific study on the effectiveness of cupping is underway, anecdotal data and historical practices indicate a wide range of potential advantages.

Types of Cupping Techniques:

Cupping therapy includes several approaches, each with its methodology and application. The most popular types are dry cupping, wet cupping, fire cupping, and moving cupping.

Dry cupping is the process of producing a vacuum in the cups without making any incisions or bloodletting.

The cups are placed in particular locations of the body and left there for a set amount of time, usually 5 to 15 minutes. This technique is frequently used to relieve pain, relax, and improve overall well-being.

Wet cupping, also known as hijama, is a more complicated procedure in which small incisions are made in the skin before putting the cups. The suction created helps draw out a little volume of blood, which is thought to eliminate toxins from the body. Wet cupping is commonly used for detoxifying and treating particular health issues.

Fire cupping uses heat to create suction in the cups. Before applying the product to the skin, a flame is momentarily put into the cup to expel air and produce a vacuum. The heat increases the suction effect, which is supposed to boost the movement of energy and blood.

Moving cupping is putting oil on the skin and utilizing cups to produce suction as they move around the body's surface. This technique is thought to increase circulation and relieve muscle tightness. The sliding cups can be used in either a linear or circular motion, depending on the therapeutic goals.

Cupping therapy is a versatile and traditional healing method that has endured the test of time. Cupping originated in numerous traditional medical systems and has evolved into a variety of treatments that address a wide range of health conditions. While cupping therapy has a long and varied history, recent research is increasingly focusing on its scientific basis and therapeutic usefulness. As our understanding of traditional therapeutic practices evolves, cupping treatment remains an intriguing topic with the potential to provide useful insights into holistic approaches to health and well-being.

CHAPTER 1
FUNDAMENTALS OF CUPPING THERAPY

Cupping therapy, an old healing method with roots in many cultures, is gaining traction in modern holistic medicine. Suction is applied to particular locations on the body to increase blood flow, relieve muscle tension, and promote general health. The core idea of cupping therapy is the belief that stagnation or imbalance of vital energy, known as "qi" in traditional Chinese medicine, causes a variety of health conditions. Cupping tries to restore qi flow by providing localized suction, which helps blood and energy circulate through the body's meridians. This therapy is profoundly ingrained in ancient medical systems such as Chinese medicine, Ayurveda, and Middle

Eastern medicine, demonstrating a common awareness of the body's energy channels and the significance of balance for maximum health.

Tools & Equipment

Cupping therapy's effectiveness and safety are heavily reliant on the tools and equipment used. Traditionally, cups were constructed of bamboo, animal horns, or glass. However, in modern practice, glass or plastic cups are more typically used due to their transparency, durability, and simplicity of sterilization. Cupping sets usually feature a variety of cup sizes to meet different body parts and treatment aims. The therapist may employ portable pumps, rubber bulbs, or fire-based methods to create suction within the cups.

The choice of equipment is determined by the therapist's preferences, the patient's condition, and the type of cupping being used.

As cupping therapy advances, new cupping sets may include silicone cups with built-in suction mechanisms, resulting in a more controlled and user-friendly experience.

<u>Cup Types Used for Cupping</u>

Cupping therapy consists of a range of cup types, each designed to serve certain therapeutic goals and accommodate diverse preferences. The most popular cup forms are basic round cups, which come in a variety of sizes to allow for versatility in use. There are also oval-shaped cups and custom-designed cups with suction valves or magnetic characteristics. Silicone cups are popular because they are flexible and easy to handle, allowing therapists to squeeze and release them for dynamic suction control. Another option is the vacuum cup, which includes a built-in pump for precise pressure control.

The cup type is determined by the therapist's competence, the patient's comfort level, and the desired therapeutic effect. Exploring the various cup alternatives in cupping therapy enables practitioners to personalize treatments to individual requirements and preferences.

Suction Methods

Suction methods in cupping therapy entail creating negative pressure within the cups to draw the skin and underlying tissues into them. This suction stimulates a therapeutic response by improving blood circulation, relaxing muscles, and facilitating the flow of vital energy.

One popular suction method is the classic fire cupping technique, which involves momentarily introducing a flame into the cup to heat the air within before placing it on the skin. As the air cools, it generates a vacuum, which pulls the skin into the cup. While fire cupping is effective, it must be used with caution to avoid burns, and safer alternatives such as rubber bulbs or handheld pump suction have been developed. The controlled use of handheld pumps allows therapists to adjust the suction intensity, making it appropriate for different levels of patient sensitivity and therapy goals. Silicone cups, with their squeezable form, provide a distinct suction approach that blends physical control with the advantages of traditional cupping therapy.

Cupping treatment is a holistic method of healing that has ancient roots but is still important in current medicine. Understanding the fundamentals of cupping, such as its definition and principles, the instruments and equipment utilized, the different types of cups accessible, and the various suction procedures, provides a thorough picture of this therapeutic practice. As cupping therapy becomes more widely recognized for its potential advantages, continuous research, and clinical investigations help to provide a more evidence-based understanding of its mechanics and applicability in a variety of healthcare settings. practitioner

CHAPTER TWO
TRADITIONAL AND MODERN APPROACHES

Cupping treatment is a therapeutic procedure that has been used for millennia, combining traditional and modern approaches. Traditional cupping practices have a rich history and cultural diversity, with popular techniques including Chinese Cupping, Hijama Cupping (Islamic Cupping), and Wet Cupping. On the other hand, modern cupping techniques have evolved to include Dry Cupping, Fire Cupping, and Vacuum Cupping. Each technique has its distinguishing features, applications, and cultural importance.

Traditional Cupping Practices

Chinese cupping has strong roots in traditional Chinese medicine (TCM), where it is said to balance the body's vital energy or Qi. Practitioners use glass or bamboo cups to produce a vacuum on the skin's surface, which promotes blood flow and addresses a variety of health issues. The suction effect is created using heat or mechanical equipment, and the therapy is commonly used to treat ailments such as pain, inflammation, and respiratory disorders. Chinese cupping has grown in popularity worldwide, and several athletes have supported it for its possible benefits in muscle healing and discomfort reduction.

Hijama Cupping, also known as Islamic Cupping, originated with the Prophet Muhammad's teachings. To remove stagnant blood and pollutants, tiny incisions are made in the skin, and suction is applied through cups. Hijama is highly respected in Islamic medicine due to its purported cleansing properties and capacity to treat a variety of illnesses. While some practitioners attribute spiritual benefits to this type of cupping, others highlight its physiological effects on circulation and overall well-being.

Wet Cupping is a type of cupping that combines suction and controlled bleeding. Practitioners start with dry cupping to establish suction on the skin, then make small incisions to allow controlled volumes of blood to flow out. This treatment is based on ancient medical traditions and is supposed to cleanse the blood, remove toxic substances, and activate the body's natural healing mechanisms. Despite its historical relevance, Wet Cupping has raised debate in modern medical circles due to sanitation concerns and the potential hazards of bloodletting.

<u>Contemporary Cupping Techniques</u>

Dry Cupping is a modern version of traditional cupping that does not require bloodletting.

 It works purely by creating a vacuum on the skin's surface with cups made of different materials, such as glass or silicone.

Dry cupping is commonly used to treat musculoskeletal disorders, promote relaxation, and improve blood circulation.

This approach is becoming increasingly popular in both Eastern and Western cultures as a non-invasive therapy with potential advantages for pain management and stress reduction.

Fire cupping is a classic technique in which heat is temporarily introduced into the cup before it is applied to the skin. The heat creates a vacuum as the cup cools, resulting in suction. Fire Cupping is renowned for its unique approach and is frequently associated with traditional Chinese medicine. Despite its historical roots, this practice has been criticized for the possible risks connected with open flames, as well as a lack of scientific data to support its effectiveness.

Vacuum Cupping, also known as suction cupping, is a modern technique that uses mechanical equipment to induce suction on the skin. This technique does not need heat or fire, making it a safer alternative to traditional fire cupping. Vacuum Cupping is adaptable and can be performed with a variety of cupping equipment, such as plastic or silicone cups coupled with suction pumps.

This method has gained appeal due to its versatility and convenience of use, making it available to a wider range of practitioners and patients.

Cupping therapy comprises a wide range of conventional and current techniques, each with its distinct qualities and applications.

The long history of traditional cupping procedures, including Chinese Cupping, Hijama Cupping, and Wet Cupping, demonstrates a wide range of cultural influences and ideas about cupping's medicinal advantages. Contemporary cupping techniques, including Dry Cupping, Fire Cupping, and Vacuum Cupping, demonstrate a development of this old therapy to satisfy the demands and preferences of both modern practitioners and patients. As cupping treatment is investigated and integrated into healthcare practices, a detailed understanding of both traditional and modern approaches will help to provide a more complete picture of this therapeutic modality.

CHAPTER 3
CUPPING POINTS AND TECHNIQUES

Cupping therapy, an ancient alternative medicine practice, involves applying cups to the skin to create suction. This therapy is based on traditional Chinese medicine (TCM) and has been practiced for centuries in numerous countries. Cupping treatment uses a variety of concepts and approaches to address specific health conditions. One critical component is identifying cupping spots and understanding the flow of qi along meridians. Cupping is used to treat a variety of ailments, including pain alleviation, detoxification, respiratory conditions, circulatory abnormalities, and skin conditions.

Meridian Points and Energy Flow: Cupping therapy is closely linked to the notion of meridians, which are energy routes in the body according to traditional Chinese medicine. These meridians are said to transport vital energy (qi) throughout the body.

Cupping points are precise spots along the meridians where cups are used to increase the flow of energy and correct imbalances. Practitioners carefully choose cupping sites based on the patient's symptoms and the underlying TCM diagnosis.

Cupping therapy works by applying cups to these meridian sites to restore qi balance, promote general well-being, and cure a variety of health ailments.

Cupping Target Areas: Choosing the right cupping target areas is critical to attaining therapeutic results.

Cupping is commonly used to target certain organs or systems in the body. For example, cupping on the back is widely used to treat respiratory disorders by targeting lung meridians. Cups can also be placed on the belly for digestive difficulties, as this area is related to the stomach and spleen meridians. Understanding the interconnection of meridians and their relationship to bodily systems helps practitioners choose the most effective target regions for cupping therapy based on an individual's health needs.

Cupping Methods for Specific Conditions: Cupping therapy uses a range of techniques, each adapted to a specific health issue. One key focus is pain management, with cupping used to reduce musculoskeletal pain and increase relaxation. The cups produce suction, which draws blood to the damaged areas, promoting healing and relieving discomfort. Cupping is also used for detoxification, which aims to remove toxins from the body. The technique is thought to improve the body's natural cleansing processes by applying cups to certain detoxification spots and facilitating the evacuation of metabolic waste.

Cupping therapy is commonly used to treat respiratory disorders like asthma, bronchitis, and coughs. The cups are precisely positioned on the back to target the lung and respiratory meridians. The cups' suction is considered to assist expand the airways, reduce inflammation, and enhance phlegm discharge. This therapy is frequently coupled with other

TCM methods to address respiratory disorders holistically, providing a more complete treatment approach.

Circulatory Disorders: Cupping therapy is used to improve blood circulation and address concerns such as inadequate flow and stagnation. Practitioners may use cups along certain meridians related to the circulatory system or to target locations with inadequate blood flow. The suction formed by the cups is thought to stimulate blood vessels, improve circulation, and aid in the evacuation of stagnant blood. Cupping therapy's ability to enhance blood flow is thought to be effective in the treatment of varicose veins and peripheral vascular disorders.

Cupping treatment is used to treat a variety of skin disorders, including eczema, acne, and cellulite.

The cups can be put into problematic areas or meridians to increase blood flow and stimulate the skin's natural healing processes. The suction formed by the cups is said to promote the discharge of toxins, reduce inflammation, and regenerate healthy skin cells. While cupping is not a stand-alone treatment for severe skin issues, it is frequently used in concert with other skincare techniques to create a more holistic therapeutic approach.

Cupping treatment includes a variety of concepts and procedures designed to promote overall well-being. Cupping points and procedures are inextricably tied to traditional

Chinese medicine ideas, particularly meridian points and energy flow.

Cupping target regions are chosen based on an understanding of meridian systems and their relationship to specific organs and bodily functions. Cupping procedures are used to treat a variety of diseases, including pain alleviation, detoxification, respiratory troubles, circulation disorders, and skin problems. The careful and targeted use of cupping therapy demonstrates its adaptability as an alternative therapeutic technique with potential advantages for a wide range of health conditions.

CHAPTER 4
PREPAREDNESS AND SAFETY MEASURES

Cupping therapy, an old healing method with roots in ancient Egyptian, Chinese, and Middle Eastern cultures, is becoming increasingly popular in modern alternative medicine.

As practitioners and receivers alike explore the therapeutic benefits of cupping, precise preparation is essential to guarantee a safe and effective session. The preliminary phase has several components, starting with a grasp of the tools and processes used.

<u>Preparing for a cupping session</u>

The preparation for a cupping session is a complex process that necessitates meticulous attention to detail.

Practitioners must ensure that the cupping equipment is in good working order, with no faults or damage. This entails thoroughly inspecting the cups, whether silicone, glass, or plastic, to avoid causing harm to the patient during therapy. Furthermore, keeping an appropriate supply of flames or suction cups, depending on the technology used, is critical for a smooth session. To achieve the intended therapeutic outcomes, practitioners must become familiar with the procedures they wish to apply, whether dry cupping, wet cupping, or fire cupping.

Understanding the patient's medical history and unique demands is an important part of session preparation. This entails a conversation between the practitioner and the patient to acquire information regarding pre-existing conditions, medications, and any concerns the individual may have.

This stage is critical for personalizing the cupping session to the patient's demands and health situation, resulting in a personalized and effective therapeutic experience.

<u>Hygiene and sanitation</u>

Maintaining a high standard of hygiene and sanitization is critical in cupping therapy to avoid infections and ensure the patient's well-being. Practitioners must follow strict cleaning measures, beginning with the sterilization of cupping equipment. Whether utilizing reusable or disposable cups, complete cleaning, and disinfection are required to remove any potential germs and pollutants. This rigorous method not only protects the patient but also maintains the professionalism and ethical standards of cupping therapy.

Beyond cup sterilization, practitioners must prioritize personal hygiene. Clean hands, adequately cleaned tools, and the use of disposable gloves help to create an aseptic atmosphere throughout the cupping session. This emphasis on sanitation is especially important while performing wet cupping, as the operation entails making micro-incisions in the skin.

To avoid infections and problems, a sterile environment must be maintained throughout this process.

<u>Patient screening and contraindications</u>

Patient screening is an essential part of cupping therapy preparation, acting as a precautionary tool to identify any contraindications or potential hazards. Thorough screening includes getting the patient's complete medical history, including current health concerns, medications, and previous experiences with cupping or alternative therapies. This information allows practitioners to make informed decisions about whether cupping is appropriate for a certain individual.

Contraindications to cupping therapy include hemophilia, pregnancy, skin infections, and certain drugs that alter blood clotting. Understanding these contraindications is critical for practitioners seeking to avoid potential consequences and protect the patient's safety. Furthermore, practitioners must be sensitive to any specific concerns or fears that the patient may have, and address them with empathy and honesty to foster trust and improve the entire therapy experience.

Safety protocols

To mitigate potential dangers and create a safe environment for both the practitioner and the patient, safety protocols must be established and followed throughout cupping therapy. These protocols cover a wide range of topics, starting with the choice of appropriate cupping procedures based on the individual's health situation and preferences. Individuals with a poor pain threshold, for example, may benefit from moderate suction cups rather than fire cupping's harsher draw.

In addition to technique selection, monitoring the duration of the cupping session is critical for avoiding side effects. Overextending the length of cupping, particularly in specific locations, might result in bruising, skin irritation, or discomfort. Practitioners must monitor the patient's response throughout the session and alter the intensity and duration accordingly to strike a balance between therapeutic advantages and potential hazards.

Cupping therapy safety protocols include emergency planning. While adverse events are uncommon, practitioners must be prepared to deal with circumstances like severe bleeding during wet cupping or unexpected reactions from patients.

A thorough approach to safety in cupping therapy includes having critical first aid supplies, knowing emergency procedures, and being able to respond quickly and calmly to unforeseen occurrences.

Cupping therapy's successful application requires rigorous preparation and adherence to safety procedures. Practitioners must traverse the complexities of equipment preparation, cleanliness requirements, patient screening, and safety measures to deliver a safe, effective, and individualized therapeutic environment.

CHAPTER 5
CLAMPING THERAPY PROTOCOLS

Cupping therapy, an old form of alternative medicine, is applying cups to the skin to create a vacuum and encourage healing. The therapy has evolved over decades and is based on traditional Chinese medicine. Cupping is thought to balance the body's essential energy (qi) and improve blood circulation. Cupping therapy techniques follow a systematic approach to assure effectiveness and safety.

<u>Standard Cupping Session Steps:</u>

To obtain the best outcomes, a conventional cupping session follows a well-defined set of stages. To evaluate whether cupping therapy is appropriate for the patient, the practitioner first assesses his or her health history and current state. Once deemed appropriate, the patient's skin is greased to allow for smooth cup movement. The cups, usually made of glass, silicone, or bamboo, are then placed on certain acupoints or affected parts of the body. The practitioner generates a vacuum inside the cups using heat or mechanical suction, causing suction pressure on the skin.

The cups stay in place for a predetermined amount of time, during which the negative pressure boosts blood flow, relieves tension, and encourages the body's natural healing processes. After the given time, the cups are removed, and the practitioner may use other techniques, such as massage or acupuncture, to boost the therapeutic effects. Throughout the session, communication between the practitioner and the patient is essential for monitoring comfort levels and adjusting therapy as necessary.

<u>Duration and frequency of sessions:</u>

The appropriate duration and frequency of cupping therapy sessions are determined by a variety of criteria, including the patient's health, treatment goals, and individual response to the therapy. A single cupping session typically lasts 15 to 30 minutes, though this might vary depending on the practitioner's method and the needs of the patient. The number of sessions varies greatly, with some people benefiting from weekly therapy and others finding monthly sessions sufficient. Chronic diseases frequently necessitate more regular sessions at first, which eventually reduce to maintenance sessions as symptoms improve. It is critical to achieve a balance between offering adequate therapeutic stimulation and allowing the body to recuperate between sessions. Determine the right time and frequency based on the severity of the problem, the patient's overall health, and their responsiveness to cupping therapy.

The practitioner must examine the treatment plan regularly to make any adjustments.

<u>Integration With Other Therapies:</u>

Cupping therapy can be combined with a variety of different therapeutic approaches to improve overall treatment outcomes. Cupping and acupuncture are frequently used together to address a variety of health conditions. Acupuncture's precision needle placement, paired with cupping's broader tissue stimulation, can generate a synergistic therapeutic impact.

Cupping therapy can also be combined with massage to increase the relaxing and tissue mobilization benefits. Physical therapists may include cupping into their rehabilitation programs to treat muscle imbalances and improve speedier injury recovery. Furthermore, cupping can supplement traditional medical therapies for certain illnesses, providing a more comprehensive approach to healthcare. When integrating cupping therapy with other modalities, healthcare professionals must collaborate and communicate effectively to ensure a comprehensive and well-coordinated treatment plan tailored to each patient's specific needs.

Cupping therapy protocols follow a methodical approach that includes typical session procedures, consideration of duration and frequency, and integration with other therapeutic modalities. Following these rules allows practitioners to maximize the therapeutic benefits of cupping while also assuring the patient's safety and comfort. This old discipline is still evolving and is now recognized as a significant supplemental therapy in modern healthcare.

CHAPTER 6
THE SCIENCE BEHIND CUPPING.

Cupping treatment, an old medical method, has acquired popularity in modern times because of its possible therapeutic effects. Cupping's science is based on its effects on the body's physiology, with a particular emphasis on the circulatory system and the fascial network. The application of cups creates a vacuum, which causes suction on the skin's surface. This suction increases blood flow and lymphatic drainage, which aids in the elimination of toxins and metabolic waste products. The negative pressure created by cupping also causes a response in the body's tissues, influencing the release of numerous biochemical mediators such as cytokines and growth factors.

These mediators are essential in the body's healing processes, helping to repair and regenerate tissues. Furthermore, cupping is thought to affect the autonomic nervous system, increasing relaxation and lowering tension.

Physiological Effects on the Body:

Cupping therapy has a variety of physiological impacts on the body, influencing various systems and improving general well-being. One of the key outcomes is improved blood circulation. Cupping creates negative pressure, which pushes blood to the skin's surface, enhancing microcirculation and oxygenation. This enhanced blood flow is supposed to help supply nutrients to cells and remove waste materials. Cupping also stimulates the lymphatic system, which promotes lymph fluid drainage and boosts the immune response. Cupping may help to remove germs and poisons from the body by stimulating lymphatic circulation. Cupping's mechanical action on the soft tissues also causes stretching, which relieves fascial limitations and improves flexibility. Furthermore, the therapy is thought to modify the activity of specific neurotransmitters, resulting in pain alleviation and relaxation.

<u>Research Studies and Clinical Evidence:</u>

While cupping therapy has a long history, recent scientific studies have aimed to prove its usefulness and understand its mechanisms. Numerous research studies and clinical trials have investigated the impact of cupping on a variety of health issues, offering information on its potential advantages.

Several researches has looked into how cupping can help with pain management, particularly in musculoskeletal problems such as neck pain, back pain, and osteoarthritis. These research findings imply that cupping could provide significant pain relief, presumably through mechanisms such as enhanced blood circulation, endorphin production, and pain perception modification. Furthermore, studies have looked into the impact of cupping on inflammatory disorders, with some finding a drop-in inflammation marker following cupping sessions. However, the variability of study designs and variations in cupping techniques make it difficult to draw firm results, emphasizing the need for more standardized research methodologies.

Cupping has also been shown in clinical studies to be effective in certain respiratory diseases.

Studies have looked into its possible benefits for asthma and chronic obstructive pulmonary disease (COPD). While the findings are encouraging, more well-designed clinical trials are needed to establish cupping as an effective supplementary therapy in respiratory care. Furthermore, researchers have looked at the psychological effects of cupping on stress, anxiety, and sadness. Preliminary research suggests that cupping may improve mental health, presumably by influencing the autonomic nervous system and releasing stress-reducing neurotransmitters. However, additional rigorous research is required to validate these findings and better understand the psychological mechanisms involved.

Despite the rising quantity of studies, determining the efficacy of cupping remains difficult due to methodological limitations, variability in cupping techniques, and the placebo effect. To improve the reliability and generalizability of findings, future studies should use bigger sample sizes, established methodologies, and stringent control groups. Furthermore, investigating personalized approaches, taking into account aspects such as patient characteristics and specific health issues, could help us gain a more nuanced knowledge of cupping therapy's therapeutic potential.

<u>Common misconceptions and myths:</u>

Cupping treatment, like many other alternative therapeutic approaches, is not immune to misinformation and falsehoods. One prevalent myth is that cupping causes permanent and ugly markings on the skin. Circular bruises or discolorations commonly linked with cupping may not indicate injury or harm. Instead, they are caused by the bursting of capillaries beneath the skin as a result of the negative pressure used during cupping. These spots, known as petechiae, usually dissolve after a few days and may not indicate serious tissue damage. Educating people on the nature of these marks is critical for reducing anxiety and fostering informed decisions about cupping therapy.

Another common misconception is that cupping therapy is a one-size-fits-all strategy. Cupping techniques vary, including dry cupping, wet cupping, and fire cupping, with each having its own set of applications and purposes.

Dry cupping creates a vacuum through suction, whereas wet cupping makes small incisions on the skin to remove a small amount of blood. Fire cupping, on the other hand, uses heat to produce a suction effect.

The cupping technique used is determined by the individual's health, preferences, and therapeutic aims. Understanding these variances is critical for both practitioners and patients seeking cupping therapy.

There is also a misperception that cupping therapy is only used in traditional Chinese medicine. While cupping has historical roots in ancient Chinese medicinal methods, it is important to understand its existence in numerous cultures throughout history, including Egyptian, Greek, and Middle Eastern traditions.

Cupping has evolved and adapted to various cultural contexts, exhibiting its adaptability and worldwide popularity. Dismissing cupping as a mere component of traditional Chinese medicine oversimplifies its profound historical and cultural importance.

Furthermore, several fallacies arise from the link of cupping therapy with pseudoscientific promises, such as detoxification or medical cures. Cupping may improve circulation, pain management, and some health conditions, but it is not a cure-all. Detoxification claims frequently lack scientific support, and individuals should view such pronouncements with skepticism. Cupping therapy should be seen as a complementary or supplemental method to standard medical care, with possible advantages recognized within a scientific framework.

Cupping therapy, which has its roots in ancient healing methods, continues to entice and captivate people seeking alternative approaches to health and well-being.

The research behind cupping focuses on its impacts on physiological processes, including circulation, lymphatic drainage, and the neurological system. Research studies and clinical evidence help us understand the potential benefits of cupping, but there are still issues with study design and consistency. Addressing common misconceptions and myths about cupping is critical for making informed decisions and encouraging a more nuanced understanding of this ancient therapeutic practice in modern circumstances.

CHAPTER 7
COMBINING CUPPING WITH OTHER HEALING PRACTICES

Cupping therapy, an ancient healing practice with thousands of years of history, has recently sparked renewed interest due to its possible therapeutic effects. Cupping therapy is unique in that it may be used with a variety of different healing modalities, providing a more holistic approach to health and wellness. When used with acupuncture, cupping produces a synergistic effect that improves the efficacy of both techniques. Acupuncture, based on traditional Chinese medicine, is the

pg. 57

insertion of tiny needles into particular places on the body to enhance energy flow. When paired with cupping, which involves applying suction to the skin's surface with cups, the two therapies work together to improve circulation, ease tension, and restore balance to the body's energy systems.

Cupping and acupuncture work together because they both aim to boost the body's vital energy or Qi. Cupping can be used before or after acupuncture sessions to prepare the body for needle stimulation or to boost the effectiveness of the needles. Cupping creates suction, which increases blood flow to the treated areas, facilitates Qi movement, and encourages the body's natural healing processes. Furthermore, the combination of cupping with acupuncture is thought to address both meridian channels and specific acupoints more thoroughly, providing a more holistic approach to treating a variety of health disorders.

Incorporating cupping therapy into massage sessions is another method that has gained popularity due to its potential to enhance the benefits of massage therapy. Massage therapy, a well-known method for inducing relaxation and relieving muscular tension, might be improved by the inclusion of cupping. Cupping, which involves strategically placing cups on the body and creating suction, helps to remove fascial limitations and enhance blood circulation. When paired with massage techniques, cupping can more effectively target specific regions of tension, resulting in a deeper and more complete release of muscle tightness.

The symbiotic link between cupping and massage is based on their common goals of increasing circulation and reducing muscular tension. Cupping's capacity to apply negative pressure to the skin lifts and separates the layers of connective tissue, allowing for enhanced blood flow and nutrient exchange. This, in turn, enhances the physical manipulation of muscles in massage therapy, allowing for a more comprehensive release of tension. Furthermore, the use of cupping in massage sessions may aid in the detoxification process by increasing the evacuation of metabolic waste products from the tissues, so adding to a general sensation of wellness.

The incorporation of cupping therapy into Western medicine symbolizes a synthesis of traditional therapeutic traditions and modern medical procedures. While cupping has ancient origins, its integration into Western medicine recognizes its promise as a supplemental therapy for a variety of illnesses. Cupping integration into Western medical settings entails collaboration between traditional cupping therapy practitioners and conventional healthcare specialists, resulting in a multidisciplinary patient care approach.

One way that cupping has been integrated into Western medicine is through its use in pain treatment. Cupping therapy has been shown in studies to help relieve musculoskeletal pain, offering it an option for patients seeking non-pharmacological interventions. By introducing cupping into pain management regimens, healthcare providers can provide patients with a complementary strategy that addresses both the symptoms and the underlying causes of pain. This integrated strategy is consistent with the greater trend in Western medicine of adopting holistic and patient-centered therapy.

Cupping therapy has also been investigated as a potential complement to standard therapies in respiratory diseases. According to research, cupping may improve lung function by increasing bronchodilation and decreasing inflammation. Cupping can help individuals with respiratory illnesses including asthma or chronic obstructive pulmonary disease (COPD) manage their symptoms and improve their overall respiratory health. This integrative approach enables a more thorough and tailored treatment strategy by recognizing the potential benefits of both traditional and Western therapy approaches.

The use of cupping therapy in other healing modalities such as acupuncture, massage therapy, and Western medicine demonstrates the ancient modality's versatility and adaptability.

The synergistic effects of combining cupping with acupuncture and massage treatment highlight the potential for improved therapeutic outcomes. Furthermore, the use of cupping in Western medicine represents a fusion of ancient and modern approaches to healthcare, offering patients a more thorough and personalized treatment experience. As researchers continue to investigate the processes and efficacy of cupping therapy, its role in integrative healthcare is expected to change, adding to the growing panorama of complementary and alternative medicine.

CHAPTER 8
CASE STUDIES AND TESTIMONIALS.

Case studies and testimonies are critical to evaluating the efficacy and effects of cupping therapy. These anecdotal experiences provide useful information on how people have experienced and profited from this alternative therapy. Examining unique cases enables practitioners and researchers to examine various illnesses and the outcomes of cupping therapy. These studies frequently demonstrate cupping's adaptability in treating a wide range of health ailments, from musculoskeletal disorders to respiratory conditions. Furthermore, they add to the current body of knowledge by providing thorough information on treatment procedures, session frequencies, and long-term outcomes. Case studies can shed light on any potential side effects or restrictions related to cupping therapy, giving a more complete knowledge of its use.

<u>Real-world Experiences and Success Stories:</u>

Real-life experiences and success stories provide a more personal and relatable look into cupping therapy. These anecdotes go beyond clinical observations and explore the subjective experiences of people who have had cupping treatments. Success stories highlight cupping's positive impact on an individual's quality of life, with a focus on improvements in physical health, emotional well-being, and general vitality. Exploring a diverse variety of success stories can provide a more nuanced picture of cupping therapy's overall advantages. These stories also serve as a source of motivation for anyone considering or undergoing cupping, instilling hope and encouragement. Examining the patterns and commonalities in success stories helps to build evidence-based procedures in cupping therapy.

Challenges Faced and Overcome:

While cupping therapy has grown in popularity, it is critical to recognize the limitations that practitioners and patients experience when implementing and experiencing this alternative treatment. Challenges can take many forms, including distrust from conventional medical practitioners, regulatory issues, and misconceptions regarding cupping. Practitioners may have difficulty integrating cupping into mainstream healthcare systems, and patients may have social stigmas or reservations about trying unorthodox therapies. Overcoming these issues necessitates a diverse approach that includes education, awareness campaigns, and coordinated efforts among healthcare professionals. Analyzing the challenges encountered and successfully overcome by practitioners and patients helps to provide a more comprehensive knowledge of the larger socio-cultural and institutional circumstances around cupping therapy.

Insights from practitioners and patients:

Both practitioners and patients contribute useful insights into the practical aspects of cupping therapy. Practitioners' experiences help to refine and evolve cupping procedures, share best practices, and solve issues that arise in clinical settings. These insights could include modifications in cupping methods, the incorporation of cupping into other therapeutic modalities, and strategies for improving patient compliance and satisfaction. Patients, on the other hand, share their preferences, expectations, and overall experiences with cupping therapy. Understanding patients' viewpoints enables practitioners to adjust therapies to specific needs, resulting in a patient-centered approach. Furthermore, patient insights contribute to the ongoing conversation between practitioners and researchers, influencing the progress of cupping treatment as a patient-friendly and culturally appropriate intervention.

Exploring case studies and testimonials, comprehending real-life experiences and success stories, appreciating the problems experienced and conquered, and learning from practitioners and patients all contribute to a thorough understanding of cupping therapy. These features offer a comprehensive overview of the efficacy, challenges, and practical consequences of adopting cupping into healthcare practices. As cupping treatment gains popularity, a detailed consideration of these principles becomes increasingly important in supporting evidence-based practices and promoting informed decision-making for both practitioners and patients looking for alternative therapeutic choices.

CHAPTER 9
CULTURAL AND ETHICAL CONSIDERATIONS

<u>Cultural perspectives on cupping:</u>

Cupping therapy has a long history that is intricately linked with various cultural perspectives around the world. Cupping, which has its roots in ancient traditions, has been adopted by many nations, each with its own set of beliefs and applications. Cupping is used in Traditional Chinese Medicine (TCM) to balance the body's vital energy, or Qi, and improve blood flow. Cupping has been used as a treatment in Middle Eastern civilizations for centuries, dating back to Prophet Muhammad's teachings. Similarly, in Ayurveda, India's traditional medicine system, cupping is regarded as an effective therapy for detoxification and dosha balance. Understanding and respecting these various cultural viewpoints is critical for practitioners providing culturally competent and empathetic cupping therapy.

The varieties of cupping utilized in different traditions reflect cultural variety. While dry cupping is widely used in Chinese and Middle Eastern cultures, wet cupping, which involves controlled bloodletting, is more frequent in Islamic traditional medicine. The subtle distinctions in cupping procedures reflect the complex tapestry of cultural beliefs and behaviors that surround this healing approach. To properly personalize cupping treatments for particular patients, practitioners must understand these cultural nuances. Furthermore, understanding the cultural significance of cupping helps practitioners build open communication and trust with their clients, which contributes to a more holistic and patient-centered approach to healthcare.

Ethical guidelines for cupping practitioners:

In the field of cupping therapy, ethical considerations are critical to ensuring patients' well-being and safety. Practitioners are guided by ethical norms that regulate their behavior and relationships with clients.

Cupping therapy requires informed permission, which is a fundamental ethical necessity. Practitioners must present patients with thorough information regarding the operation, potential risks, and projected outcomes so that they can make educated healthcare decisions. Furthermore, practitioners must respect patient autonomy by ensuring that patients can decline or terminate cupping treatments at any time.

Confidentiality is another important ethical consideration in cupping therapy. Practitioners must protect the privacy and confidentiality of patient information while providing a secure and confidential setting for talks and treatments. This is especially crucial considering the sensitivity of health-related information, as well as the potential cultural or societal stigmas associated with specific illnesses.

Practitioners must also follow the principle of nonmaleficence, ensuring that cupping procedures are performed with extreme caution to avoid injury to the patient. This includes maintaining current with best practices, using sanitary equipment, and understanding contraindications to cupping therapy. Furthermore, practitioners have an ethical obligation to continually examine and improve their abilities, as well as engage in ongoing professional development, to deliver the best possible treatment.

<u>Cultural Sensitivity and Cupping Therapy:</u>

Cultural awareness is essential in the practice of cupping therapy, as practitioners must be aware of their patients' different backgrounds, beliefs, and values.

It entails recognizing and respecting the cultural settings that influence people's conceptions of health and wellness.

One important part of cultural sensitivity in cupping therapy is acknowledging that patients' comfort levels with touch, exposure, or discussions about their bodies may differ depending on cultural norms.

Effective communication is a key component of cultural sensitivity in cupping therapy. Practitioners must be adept at managing linguistic and cultural gaps to develop clear and open lines of communication with their patients.

This involves the ability to speak in a culturally appropriate manner, actively listen to patient's issues, and change communication approaches to create trust and understanding.

Understanding cultural nuances includes nutrition and lifestyle factors. For example, food habits may be inextricably linked to cultural or religious customs, altering the body's response to cupping therapy. Practitioners must understand these linkages to make individualized recommendations that are appropriate for their patients' cultural backgrounds.

Furthermore, cultural sensitivity includes understanding the potential influence of cupping therapy on mental health. Some patients may have cultural beliefs that influence their mental health; thus practitioners must approach mental health discussions with empathy and cultural competence. This includes being aware of any cultural taboos or sensitivities related to mental health and dealing with them sensitively and respectfully.

Cultural and ethical factors are essential to offering effective and responsible cupping therapy. Practitioners must navigate the complex tapestry of cultural ideas around cupping, follow ethical rules to maintain patient safety and acquire cultural sensitivity to interact with varied patient communities. By taking these factors into account, cupping therapy can be given in a way that respects individual values, builds trust, and improves patients' overall health and well-being.

CHAPTER 10
FUTURE TRENDS AND INNOVATION

Cupping treatment, an old therapeutic method, has seen a boom in popularity in recent years. As the need for alternative and complementary therapies grows, the future of cupping therapy seems promising in terms of evolving procedures and equipment. Cupping technique innovations are likely to focus on increasing efficacy, decreasing side effects, and giving a more personalized approach to therapy. Researchers and practitioners alike are looking at new ways to improve conventional cupping techniques by incorporating technological breakthroughs and modern medical expertise.

The creation of customized cups and equipment is one example of cupping therapy innovation. Traditional cupping uses glass or plastic cups that are heated and put to the skin to create a suction effect. However, continued study and technology improvements have resulted in the development of more complex cupping tools. Manufacturers are looking at materials that improve suction capabilities, and hygiene, and allow for greater control over the therapeutic process. This advancement in technology is intended to make cupping therapy more accessible, efficient, and user-friendly for both practitioners and patients.

Advancements in cupping techniques include not only the equipment employed but also the methods of application. The use of dynamic cupping, in which cups are moved across the skin, is gaining popularity due to its potential benefits in improving circulation and addressing specific areas of concern. Furthermore, improvements in cupping massage techniques, which combine cupping therapy with manual massage, are being investigated for their synergistic effects in improving overall wellness.

<u>Ongoing Research and Development</u>

As cupping therapy becomes more widely recognized as a legitimate supplementary treatment, research into its mechanics, efficacy, and possible uses intensifies. Ongoing studies are looking at the physiological and psychological consequences of cupping to provide evidence-based support for its usage in a variety of medical disorders. Researchers are looking at the effects of cupping therapy on inflammation, blood circulation, pain management, and stress reduction.

One area of interest in cupping research is its impact on musculoskeletal problems. Cupping therapy is being studied to see if it can help with injury healing, muscular discomfort, and joint mobility. The scientific community is also looking into the potential anti-inflammatory effects of cupping, specifically the release of cytokines and other indicators involved in the body's inflammatory response.

Aside from musculoskeletal uses, researchers are investigating the benefits of cupping therapy on respiratory disorders like asthma and chronic obstructive pulmonary disease (COPD). Preliminary studies indicate that cupping may improve lung function and respiratory symptoms, but further study is needed to determine its efficacy and safety in these settings.

Cupping therapy's psychological components are also being investigated, with studies looking into its ability to reduce stress, anxiety, and sadness. Mental health researchers are interested in the relaxation induced by cupping, as well as the potential physiological impacts on the neurological system.

Potential future applications

The prospective applications of cupping therapy in the future go beyond its traditional usage. As researchers continue to identify the therapeutic mechanisms and benefits of cupping, new applications emerge. One such area is the incorporation of cupping therapy into mainstream healthcare, which includes the formulation of guidelines for its usage in conjunction with traditional medical therapies.

Cupping therapy is becoming increasingly popular as a complementary treatment for chronic illnesses such as fibromyalgia, arthritis, and neurological problems. Cupping is currently being studied to see if it can complement existing medical procedures, giving patients more alternatives for symptom management and enhancing their overall quality of life.

Cupping therapy is regarded as a wellness activity in the field of preventive healthcare, helping to maintain overall health and prevent the advent of specific illnesses.

Proponents say that regular cupping sessions can improve circulation, immunological function, and overall well-being, which aligns with holistic health beliefs.

Furthermore, the prospective uses of cupping therapy in sports medicine are gaining popularity. Athletes and sports professionals are investigating the use of cupping to increase recovery, minimize muscular fatigue, and boost athletic performance. As proof of the benefits of cupping in sports-related contexts grows, it may become more commonly acknowledged in the athletic world.

In dermatology, cupping treatment is being studied for its potential to treat skin problems such as acne, eczema, and psoriasis. Preliminary research suggests that cupping may alter skin microcirculation and immunological responses, opening the door to its usage as a supplemental strategy in dermatological care.

CONCLUSION

Cupping therapy, which has its roots in ancient healing practices, is resurging and evolving in today's healthcare scene. The future of cupping therapy seems promising, with continual advancements in techniques and equipment broadening its potential applications.

The incorporation of technical developments into cupping tools, as well as the development of dynamic cupping procedures, demonstrate the ancient practice's adaptation to modern healthcare needs.

Continuous research and development are critical in developing the scientific basis for cupping therapy.

 Studies looking into its benefits on musculoskeletal disorders, pulmonary health, and psychological well-being add to the expanding body of evidence supporting its usage in a variety of settings. Cupping therapy's potential applications in mainstream healthcare, preventive medicine, sports medicine, and dermatology suggest that it is becoming more widely used in medical procedures.

While cupping therapy shows promise, it is critical to approach its use with a balanced mindset. Rigorous scientific research is required to determine its efficacy, safety, and best practices. As cupping therapy gains popularity, collaboration between traditional practices and evidence-based medicine is critical to ensuring its safe integration into comprehensive healthcare systems.

the future of cupping therapy is dynamic, with ongoing research, technical developments, and a growing number of potential uses. As the discipline evolves, practitioners, researchers, and healthcare professionals must collaborate to evaluate its efficacy, investigate new avenues, and contribute to the integration of cupping treatment into holistic and patient-centered healthcare systems.

www.ingramcontent.com/pod-product-compliance
Lightning Source LLC
Chambersburg PA
CBHW060751260726

48660CB00002B/579